GREEN DIET

Quick and Easy Vegan Recipes

The Health Buff

The information provided in this book is designed to provide helpful information on the subjects discussed. The author's books are only meant to provide the reader with the basics knowledge of the topic in question, without any warranties regarding whether the reader will, or will not, be able to incorporate and apply all the information provided. Although the writer will make his best effort share her insights, the topic in question is a complex one, and each person needs a different timeframe to fully incorporate new information. Neither this book, nor any of the author's books constitute a promise that the reader will learn anything within a certain timeframe.

Table Of Contents

Introduction

Veganism is the practice of abstaining or cutting back from the use of animal products, specifically in diet, and an philosophy that rejects the commodity status of animals. Vegan is the person that follows this kind of lifestyle.

Vegan diets are mostly based on grains, legumes, fruits, vegetables, edible mushrooms and nuts. Meat alternatives are usually based on soybeans (tofu) that are in the form of veggie sausage and burgers.

Vegans also eat many of the same common and familiar everyday foods such as a green salad, spaghetti, and chips and salsa which just about everyone eats that are usually in plant-based ingredients.

While some people easily go from eating meat to vegan right away, others struggle with their new commitment, or choose to go vegetarian first and then slowly trim eggs and dairy. There's no right or wrong way to do it, but you may want to learn about what's worked for other people. Whatever way you want to do it, keep your goals in mind and remember why you are choosing to adopt a vegan diet.

Continue to enjoy your favorite desserts like cakes and your comfort food, soup and healthy meals (most probably all your favorite dishes) in a vegan friendly way.

Here are some delish vegan recipes that are quick and easy to prepare and will make you choose to go on this lifestyle.

HEALTHY BREAKFAST RECIPES

Shamrock Breakfast Sandwich

Ingredients:

For Patty:

- 1 vegan sausage patty
- dash chipotle powder
- dash fine black pepper
- dash seasoned salt
- rub of veggie oil

Kale saute:

- 2 cups kale, torn
- 1/2 tsp truffle infused oil
- 1 tsp extra virgin olive oil
- dash fine pepper
- 2 Tbsp raw pumpkin seeds
- a few dashes seasoned salt
- 1/2 shallot, thinly sliced

Jalapeno Mayo:

- 1 1/2 Tbsp Vegenaise
- 1/2 tsp dried jalapeno
- dash chipotle powder
- dash seasoned salt
- 1 Tbsp sweet green juice for color/thinning (or use citrus juice)

- sliced avocado, lemon juice rubbed (2-4 slices)
- 1 English Muffin, toasted

Reminder: You can reduce the oil used in the cooking process to lighten the total calories if desired. You can easily cook the components without using any oil and just a few splashes of water.

Instruction:

1. Add a drizzle of oil to a saute pan. Turn heat to high. Add in the chopped shallot. Cook for until shallot starts to brown. Pour shallot and oil into small bowl then set aside.
2. Keep heat on high and lay your vegan sausage patty in the pan. I use the kind that comes in tube and you can press out into whatever thicknes, size you'd like. Cooks super fast. Well seasoned, but I add a few extra spices. While cooking, add spices to both sides of patty. Add a drizzle of oil if desired. The patties are naturally fat free, but I add a splash of oil to saute. Cook 1-2 minutes on each side - until edges brown. Remove hot patty and set aside.
3. Add all the kale saute ingredients to the warm pan. Cover with lid while the kale cooks.steams for about one minute. You just want to wilt the kale and infuse it with some flavor. Turn off the

heat and then transfer wilted kale to bowl. Toss the shallot with the kale and pepitas.
4. Mix together the vegan jalapeno mayo.
5. Assemble! Spread the vegan jalapeno sauce/mayo on the inside of each toasted English muffin. Add sliced avocado, patty, then top with plenty of the kale mixture. Close sandwich with top muffin and serve warm!
6. Side of citrus, kale, grape, mint, pineapple, soy green juice is lovely.

Matcha Breakfast Pizza

Ingredients:

- 4 tbsp buckwheat flour
- dash pink salt
- 1 tsp baking powder
- 1/2 tsp cinnamon
- 1 tsp matcha
- 1 egg
- 2 tbsp maple syrup/raw honey
- 75ml almond/oat milk
- 1 banana
- 2 tsp coconut oil
- 2 tbsp organic whole milk yoghurt/coconut yoghurt
- goji berries, seeds and bee pollen, to top

Instruction:

1. Mix the buckwheat flour, salt, baking powder, cinnamon and matcha in a baking bowl so well combined.
2. Crack egg and squeeze in a tablespoon of the maple/honey and whisk well.
3. Slowly add in the milk and keep whisking until it results in a thick pancake consistency. If it's too runny, add more flour and if it's too thick – add more milk!

4. Heat up 1tsp coconut oil on a medium heat in a
   pan and pour in the whole mix. Let it cook
   through until bubbles start to appear on the top
   and carefully use a spatula to turn around and
   cook on the other side. This won't take too long
   – around 4 minutes all in all!
5. While you're waiting, heat up the other
   teaspoon coconut oil in a separate pan and
   add in the chopped banana with a pinch of
   cinnamon and sautee for a minute until soft
   and 'caramelly.'
6. Put to the side and serve the pancake up on a
   plate, slather with the yoghurt and top with the
   goji berries, bee pollen, seeds, banana and the
   remaining maple syrup. Dig in!

French Toasts

Ingredients:

- 5 slices bread
- 1 cup of non-dairy milk
- 1 tablespoon nutritional yeast flakes
- 2 tablespoons whole wheat flour
- 1 teaspoon cinnamon
- Maple syrup or raw honey, for topping

Instruction:

1. Mix non-dairy milk, yeast, whole wheat flour and cinnamon in a mixing bowl.
2. Place the slices of bread in a container with sides.
3. Pour the mixture over the bread, then lift of flip the bread over to make sure both sides are evenly coated.
4. Heat oil in a pan over medium heat.
5. Place the bread slices onto the pan then cook until golden brown. Flip over the other side until it is golden brown. Make sure that both sides are properly cooked.
6. For topping, drizzle maple syrup or raw honey on top of bread.

Breakfast Muffins with Blueberry

Ingredients:

- 2 cups of flour
- 1 cup of non-dairy milk
- 1 tbsp. apple cider vinegar
- ¼ cup of ground flax seed
- 1 ½ tsp baking soda
- ¼ tsp sea salt
- 1 tsp ground cinnamon
- ¼ cup of olive oil
- ½ cup of maple syrup
- 1 tsp pure vanilla extract
- ½ tsp almond extract
- 1 ½ cup of blueberries

Instruction:

1. Preheat the oven to 375 0F for 15 minutes.
2. Lightly grease a muffin tin.
3. Grind flax seeds in a medium bowl, combine flour, baking soda, salt, ground flax seeds, cinnamon and salt together.
4. In a small bowl, combine the maple syrup, milk, oil, vanilla extract, almond extract, and vinegar.
5. Mix well. Add the ingredients to the wet ingredients and stir together.
6. Stir in the blueberries.
7. Fill the muffin tins half full.

8.   Bake until golden brown color and a knife placed in the center of the muffin comes out clean (approximately 20 minutes).
9.   Remove from the oven and let it cool. Serve and enjoy.

Blueberry Peach Oatmeal

Ingredients:

- 1 1/3 cups water
- 2/3 cup regular oats
- 1 cup almond milk
- 1/2 tsp vanilla extract
- 1/2 cup blueberries
- 1/2 cup peaches
- Pinch of salt
- 1/2 tsp cinnamon
- 1/8th tsp nutmeg
- 1 tbsp. Sugar

Instruction:

1. Place the water and salt in a medium sized pot and bring to a boil. Add the oats and almond milk over medium heat.
2. Cook for about 5 minutes.
3. Add the sugar, nutmeg, cinnamon and vanilla extract and heat for another 5-7 minutes, stirring frequently.
4. Stir in the peaches and blueberries.
5. Pour into a bowl and serve.

Fruity Tutty Oatmeal

Ingredients:

- 1⁄2 cup of oatmeal
- 1⁄2 cup apple juice, refrigerated
- 1⁄2 cup of water
- 1 small apple, diced
- 3 pcs of prunes, diced
- 3 pcs of apricots, dehydrated, dried & diced
- 4 pecans, diced
- 1⁄4 tsp. cinnamon

Instruction:

1. In a small sauce pan, combine together the apple juice and water then bring to a boil.
2. Add in half cup of oatmeal, approximately a minute.
3. The moment it's cooked as per the directions mentioned on the box, remove it from the heat and let it stand for couple of minutes to cool a little and thicken.
4. Add in the pecans, cinnamon and the fruit pieces; as you're adding in, don't forget to stir and don't let them stick together.
5. To preserve more of vitamins, wait till the oatmeal is cool then add in the fruits. Serve and enjoy.

Morning Tacos

Ingredients:

- 1 cooked sweet potato
- 3 corn tortillas
- ½ cup black beans, cooked
- ½ cup kale, cooked
- 2 green onions, sliced
- 1 dash garlic powder
- 1/2 cup vegan salsa
- 2 table spoons nutritional yeast
- 3 tablespoons guacamole

Instruction:

1. Heat each side of tortillas of 2 minutes.
2. Mash sweet potato with a fork, add beans, greens, green onions, garlic powder, salsa, nutritional yeast, and guacamole as filling for tortillas.
3. Add filling to center of tortillas. Serve.

Vegan Waffles

Ingredients:

- 2 tbsp. flax seed meal
- 1 cup of rolled oats
- 1 3/4 cups of non-dairy milk
- 1/2 cup all-purpose flour
- 1/2 cup whole wheat flour
- 2 tbsp. melted coconut oil
- 4 tsp baking powder
- 1 tsp pure vanilla extract
- 1 tbsp. maple syrup
- ½ tsp salt
- ½ cup of water

Instructions:

1. Preheat waffle iron.
2. Stir water and flax seed meal together in a small bowl and allow to stand for 10 minutes so that the gel can be set.
3. Blend oats in a blender into a flour-like consistency. Add flax seed mixture, non-dairy milk, all-purpose flour, whole wheat flour, melted coconut oil, baking powder, vanilla extract, maple syrup, and salt to oats; blend until batter is just mixed.
4. Add 1/2 cup batter into preheated waffle iron.

5. Cook the waffles until golden brown for 5
    minutes. Serve.

Quinoa Porridge with Cinnamon

Ingredients:

- 1/2 cup quinoa
- 1/4 tsp ground cinnamon
- 1 1/2 cups of almond milk
- 1/2 cup of water
- 2 tbsp. brown sugar
- 1 tsp pure vanilla extract
- A pinch of salt

Instruction:

1. Heat a saucepan over medium heat.
2. Add the quinoa and cinnamon, stirring frequently, about 3 minutes.
3. Pour the almond milk, water, vanilla and stir in the brown sugar and salt.
4. Bring to a boil, cook over low heat until the porridge is thick and grains are tender, about 25 minutes. Add water as needed.

SUMPTOUS

LUNCH

VEGAN

DISHES

Tasty Tempeh and Rice

Ingredients:

- 4 ounces tempeh, cut into 1/4-inch pcs
- 1 tbsp. soy sauce
- 1 tbsp. maple syrup
- 1 tsp rice vinegar
- 1 clove garlic, minced
- 1/4 cup tahini
- 1 tbsp. miso
- 2 tsp lemon juice
- 2 tsp grated ginger
- 1/4 cup of warm water
- 3 cups kale cut into 1/2-inch pcs
- 2 cups of cooked rice
- 1/2 cup sauerkraut
- 1 avocado, sliced
- 1 tsp sesame seeds

Instructions:

1. To marinate the tempeh:
2. Mix soy sauce, maple syrup, rice vinegar, and garlic altogether.
3. Place tempeh in a shallow dish, pour marinade over, and turn to coat.
4. Let marinate for at least 20 minutes or as long as overnight in the refrigerator.

5. To make the dressing:
6. Mix tahini, miso, lemon juice, and ginger into a creamy paste in a small bowl. Gradually stir in warm water to achieve the consistency of the sauce.
7. To make the kale, fill a pot with about 1 inch of water and place a steamer basket inside.
8. Bring to a boil. Put kale in basket and cover then steam for about 5 minutes until tender but slightly crisp. To finish, cook the marinated tempeh in a lightly oiled skillet over medium heat for a few minutes on each side until golden brown. Halfway through cooking, pour the remaining marinade over tempeh.
9. Divide the steamed kale between two bowls. Place brown rice on top. Then arrange tempeh, sauerkraut and avocado on top. Sprinkle with sesame seeds. Serve with dressing on the side. Enjoy.

Soybean (Tofu) Salad

Ingredients:

- 1 tsp. basil
- 1⁄4 cup of each green & red pepper
- 1 package tofu
- 1⁄2 cup onion, diced
- 1 tsp. cumin
- 1⁄2 cup vegan mayonnaise
- 1 tsp. parsley
- 4 pcs of pita pockets

Instructions:

1. Cut the tofu into cubes and fry until golden brown, for few minutes.
2. Mix tofu with onions, mayo, seasonings (any of your choice) and peppers. Depending on your liking, you may add more or less quantity mayo to the salad.
3. Use a pita pocket to serve.

Sweet Potato Casserole

Ingredients:

- Medium sized sweet potatoes, cut in large pieces
- 1 1/2 tbsp. vegan butter
- 1 1/2 tbsp. coconut oil
- 2 1/2 tbsp. maple syrup
- 1 tsp vanilla extract
- 3/4 tsp cinnamon
- 1/8 tsp ground nutmeg
- 1/2 tsp salt
- For toppings:
- 1 cup of rolled oats
- 1 1/3 cups chopped pecan halves
- 1/3 cup of almond flour
- 1 tsp cinnamon
- 1/4 tsp salt
- 2 tbsp. coconut oil
- 2 tbsp. vegan butter, melted
- 2 1/2 tbsp. maple syrup

Instructions:

1. Peel and cut sweet potatoes into large pieces.
2. Place into a large pot and cover with water with a pinch of salt and bring water to a boil.
3. Add sweet potatoes to the pot and cook for 15 minutes.

4. Drain the sweet potatoes. Preheat oven to 375°F.
5. Lightly grease a casserole dish and set aside.
6. Now for the topping:
7. Blend the oats in a blender or food processor. In a medium bowl, stir together the pecans, oats, almond flour, cinnamon, and salt.
8. Pour the melted coconut oil, melted vegan butter, and maple syrup. Stir together.
9. Put the sweet potatoes into a large bowl and mash them.
10. Add the vegan butter and coconut oil until smooth.
11. Stir in the maple syrup, vanilla, cinnamon, nutmeg, and salt.
12. Place sweet potato mixture into a casserole dish Sprinkle the crumble topping all over the sweet potato mixture. Bake at 375°F for 20-25 minutes.
13. Let it cool and serve.

Classic Split-Pea Soup

Ingredients:

- 1 pound dried green split peas
- 6 cups of water
- 3 pcs carrots, diced
- 3 pcs celery stalks, diced
- 1 medium potato, peeled and diced
- 1 small yellow onion, diced
- 1 bay leaf
- Ground black pepper
- 1½ tsp minced garlic – 3 cloves
- 5 vegetable bouillon cubes

Ingredients:

1. Put all the split peas, water, carrots, celery, potato, onion, garlic, bouillon cubes, and bay leaf in a slow cooker; mix well.
2. Cover and cook on low heat for 6 to 8 hours.
3. Remove the bay leaf and season with pepper. Serve.

Soybean (Tofu) and Quinoa Salad

Ingredients:

- ¾ tsp salt (divided)
- 2 minced garlic cloves
- 3 tbsp. extra-virgin olive oil
- ¼ cup of lemon juice
- ½ cup fresh parsley, chopped
- ½ cup fresh mint, chopped
- ¼ tsp fresh ground black pepper
- 1 diced yellow bell pepper
- 1 cup halves grape tomatoes
- 1 cup diced cucumber
- 8oz pack of baked, smoked tofu -diced
- 1 cup rinsed quinoa
- 2 cups of water

Instructions:

1. Boil the water in a saucepan with half a teaspoon of salt in it.
2. Add the quinoa and boil. Turn the heat down and simmer for 15 to 20 minutes until the water is absorbed. Spread the quinoa over a baking sheet and let it cool for ten minutes.
3. Whisk the garlic, oil, lemon juice, quarter teaspoon salt and the pepper in a large bowl.
4. Add the cooled quinoa and the rest of the ingredients. Toss the mixture well and serve.

Vegan Squash Salad

Ingredients:

- 3 cups of butternut squash in cubes
- 1 tbsp. Dijon mustard
- 2 tbsp. balsamic vinegar
- 2 tbsp. lemon juice
- 3 oz. feta cheese, crumbled
- 2 tbsp. olive oil
- Salt and pepper to taste
- 1 tsp dried oregano
- 2 tbsp. sliced almonds
- 2 tbsp. chopped cilantro

Instructions:

1. Place the squash cubes in a baking tray and drizzle them with 2 tablespoons olive oil.
2. Sprinkle with salt, pepper and dried oregano.
3. Bake them at 375F for 30 minutes or until they start to look caramelized. Transfer them in a large bowl and stir in the sliced almonds and chopped cilantro.
4. To make the dressing, mix the mustardwith the balsamic vinegar and lemon juice. Pour the dressing over the warm squash and mix gently.
5. Place the salad on a platter and top with crumbled feta before serving.

6. Getpan, warm the seasoned zoodles over medium-high heat. Cook them for 1 to 2 minutes. Add the marinara and continue cooking for 1 more minute.

7. Plate the zoodles next to the chicken then serve immediately.

Simple and Easy Tofu Peanut Wrap

Ingredients:

- 8 inch whole wheat flour tortilla
- 2oz baked seasoned tofu, thinly sliced
- ¼ cup red bell pepper, sliced
- 1 tbsp. Thai peanut sauce
- 8 snow peas, thinly sliced

Ingredients:

1. Spread the peanut sauce on the tortilla.
2. Place the rest of the ingredients in the middle, fold the sides over and roll up.

Vegan Rice Stew

Ingredients:

- 1 cup brown rice
- 1 cup baby corn, sliced
- 1 cup of green beans
- 1 cup of green beans, chopped
- 2 cups of water
- ½ cup of coconut milk
- 2 tbsp. olive oil
- 1 finely chopped shallot
- 2 garlic cloves, chopped
- 2 carrots, sliced
- ½ teaspoon cumin powder
- 1 pinch chili powder
- 4 tablespoons chopped cilantro
- Salt, pepper to taste

Instructions:

1. Heat the skillet over medium flame and stir in the shallot and garlic.
2. Sauté for 2 minutes.
3. Stir in all the vegetables and the riceand sauté for 5 more minutes.
4. Pour in the water and coconut milk then add the cumin powder and chili.

5. Lower the heat and cover the skillet with a lid. Cook for 20-30 minutes until all the liquid has been absorbed and the veggies are tender.
6. Remove from heat and add salt and pepper then stir in the chopped cilantro.
7. Serve it warm.

Vegan Mushroom Soup

Ingredients:

- 3/4 cup of mushrooms, sliced
- 1 tsp dried thyme
- 3 cups of vegetable broth
- 2 bay leaves
- 2 tbsp. gluten-free soy sauce
- 6 tbsp. cornstarch
- 1/4 cup of cold water
- 3 cups coconut milk
- salt and ground black pepper to taste
- 1 tbsp. olive oil
- 1 large onion, diced

Instructions:

1. Heat olive oil in a large pot over medium heat.
2. Cook and stir onions until they start to soften, about 5 minutes. Add mushrooms and thyme; stir until fragrant, about 5 minutes.
3. Stir in broth, bay leaves, and soy sauce. Bring soup to a boil.
4. Whisk cornstarch and water together in a small bowl; pour into soup and stir well to incorporate. Reduce heat and simmer soup until it starts to thicken, about 10 minutes.

5. Add coconut milk, salt, and black pepper.
    Simmer just until coconut milk is heated, about
    4 minutes.

LIGHT AND EASY DINNER RECIPES

Vegan Angel Hair Pasta Primavera

Ingredients:

- 3 tbsp olive oil
- 1 onion, diced
- 3 cloves garlic, minced
- 1 tbsp dried basil
- 6 tbsp flour
- 3 cups soy milk
- 1/4 cup nutritional yeast
- 1 small head broccoli, cut into florets
- 1 medium carrot, sliced
- 1/2 pound sliced fresh mushrooms
- 1 cup frozen peas, thawed
- salt and pepper to taste
- 1 pound angel hair pasta

Instructions:

1. Heat the olive oil in a large pan in medium heat. Add in the diced onion, and the garlic and basil and allow to heat until the onion becomes translucent, about 5-7 minutes. Next, stir in the flour to make a thick paste.
2. Slowly add the soy milk, stirring constantly. Stir in the nutritional yeast, then cook over low heat just until the mixture thickens.

3. In a separate pan, using a vegetable steamer, steam the broccoli florets and the sliced carrots just until barely tender, then add them into the white sauce along with the mushrooms and thawed frozen peas.
4. Add salt and pepper to taste, then cook on low heat until fully heated while stirring often.
5. Cook the angel hair pasta according to package directions, then serve the pasta primavera sauce over the prepared pasta.
6. Enjoy your healthy vegetarian and vegan pasta primavera!

Three Bean Pasta with Creamy Spinach Sauce

Ingredients:

- 1 tablespoon olive oil
- 1 large onion, sliced
- 2 cloves garlic, crushed
- 1 red bell pepper, chopped
- 1 teaspoon dried oregano
- 1 15 ounce can chopped tomatoes, or 2 cups chopped fresh tomatoes
- 1/2 cup cooked red kidney beans
- 1/2 cup cooked navy beans
- 1/2 cup cooked chickpeas
- Salt and pepper to taste
- 1 cup small pasta tubes
- 2 tablespoons margarine
- 4 tablespoons flour
- 2 cups soy milk
- 1/2 teaspoon grated nutmeg
- 1 1/2 cups finely chopped raw spinach

Instructions:

1. Heat the oil in a large saucepan over medium heat. Lightly cook the onion, garlic, and pepper until the vegetables are soft, about 8 minutes.

2. Add the oregano, tomatoes, beans, and chickpeas. Season to taste with salt and pepper. Cover the saucepan and simmer for 20 minutes.
3. Prepare the pasta according to package directions. Drain water on pasta and add it to the cooked bean mixture and place this mixture in a shallow serving dish.
4. To make the sauce, heat the margarine in a medium saucepan over medium heat. Stir in the flour and gradually add the soy milk. Let it simmer, while stirring constantly, and cook for 2 to 3 minutes, then season with the nutmeg and salt and pepper.
5. Steam the spinach in 2 tablespoons of water for 5 minutes. Drain thoroughly and add to the sauce. Stir until well blended.
6. Pour sauce over the bean mixture and serve immediately.

Bok Choy and Shiitake Mushroom Stir-Fry

Ingredients:

- 3-4 cloves minced garlic
- 1 cup shiitake mushrooms, sliced OR 1/2 cup sliced shiitake mushrooms and 1/2 cup sliced button mushrooms
- 2 tsp canola oil
- 1 tbsp soy sauce (gluten-free)
- 1 bok choy, chopped (or 2-3 baby bok choy if you prefer)
- 5-6 scallions, sliced
- 1/4 cup vegetable broth
- 2 tsp fresh ginger, minced or grated
- 2 tsp sesame oil
- 2 tbsp sesame seeds (optional)

Instructions:

1. Sautee the garlic and mushooms in oil for 3 to 5 minutes then add in the soy sauce, the bok choy and scallions, and cook for a few more minutes.
2. Lower heat to medium and add vegetable broth and ginger. Simmer for about 3 - 5 minutes.
3. Finally, stir in the sesame oil and the optional sesame seeds and remove from heat.

4. Serve bok choy and mushroom stir-fry hot on rice, quinoa, noodles (with a little bit of sauce) or just enjoy it as is as a simple vegetable side dish.

Or, add in some fried or baked tofu to add protein and make it a main dish.

Veggie Stir-fry in Lemon Ginger Sauce

Ingredients:

- 3 Tbsp soy sauce
- 3 Tbsp fresh lemon or lime juice
- 1 Tbsp sesame oil
- 2 tsp fresh grated ginger
- 2 Tbsp canola oil, safflower oil, or other high-heat cooking oil
- 1 cup chopped cauliflower
- 1 cup chopped broccoli
- 2 carrots, sliced thin
- 1 small onion, chopped
- 1 green bell pepper, sliced
- 1 cup snow peas
- 1 cup sliced mushrooms
- 2 green onions (scallions), chopped
- 1/2 cup bean sprouts (optional)

Instructions:

1. Beat together the soy sauce, sesame oil, lemon or lime juice, and ginger then set aside.
2. In a large skillet or wok, stir-fry the cauliflower, broccoli, carrots, onion, and bell pepper in canola oil or safflower oil, stirring frequently.

3. After two minutes add the snow peas,
   mushrooms, bean sprouts, green onions and
   soy sauce mixture, stirring together to mix well.
4. Continue to stir frequently until the vegetables
   are cooked but still crunchy, another 2-3
   minutes.
5. Serve alongside some plain white rice topped
   with all the extra sauce.

Veggie Beef and Broccoli Chinese Stir-Fry Chow Mein

Ingredients:

- 1 package store-bought beef substitute (try gardein brand "beefless tips")
- 1/2 medium red onion, sliced thin
- 10 shiitake mushrooms, chopped
- 1/2 medium head broccoli, chopped into bite-sized florets
- 1 red bell pepper, diced (seeds removed)
- 1/2 cup black bean garlic sauce
- 1 bag (300g) chow mein noodles
- 3 tbsp canola oil (or other neutral oil)
- 1 green onion (scallions), chopped small
- salt and pepper, to taste

Instruction:

1. First, prepare the chow mein noodles. Bring about 4 cups of salted water to a boil and cook the noodles until tender, following the cooking instructions on the bag.
2. In a medium sautee pan, heat a bit of canola oil, and brown the beef substitute on all sides until browned and crisped. Add the onions and mushrooms, and heat for another 3-5 minutes.

3. Next, add the black bean sauce, 1/2 cup water, and the broccoli and red bell pepper. Cover the pan, and allow to heat for just a minute. Uncover, and bring to a simmer. Allow to heat, stirring frequently, until the sauce has reduced by about half.

4. For serving, top the prepared chow mein noodles with the vegetarian "beef" and broccoli mixture, and garnish with chopped green onions.

Cheesy Veggie Risotto

Ingredients:

- 3 tablespoons olive oil
- 8 cups vegetable broth
- 2 cups arborio rice
- dash salt (to taste)
- dash pepper (to taste)
- 2/3 cup parmesan (freshly grated)

Instructions:

1. In a large pan, heat the olive oil and add the arborio rice. Stir constantly, and let the rice to cook for 3 to 4 minutes.
2. Add about a half cup of the vegetable broth to the rice, stirring frequently.
3. When most of the liquid has absorbed, add another half cup of broth. Continue adding broth, a little at a time until the rice is cooked for at least 20 minutes.
4. Remove from heat and stir in the parmesan until it has thoroughly melted.
5. Add salt and pepper to taste. Sprinkle with additional cheese if desired.

Vegan Pumpkin Risotto

Ingedients:

- 1 onion, diced
- 1 tbsp. olive oil
- 2 cups arborio (risotto) rice
- 1 cup white wine
- 4 cups vegetable broth
- 1 cup canned pumpkin
- 1 tsp. fresh ginger, grated or minced
- 1 tsp nutmeg
- 1 tbsp. chopped fresh basil
- 1 tbsp. vegan margarine or butter
- Salt and pepper to taste

Instructions

1. Sautee the onion in the olive oil on medium heat for 3 to 5 minutes, or until the onion is soft. Next, add in the rice. Let it cook, stirring, for a minute or two, just to lightly toast the rice, and being carefully that it doesn't burn. Slowly add in the white wine.

2. After that, start to add the vegetable broth, 1/2 cup each time. Allow the moisture to cook off before adding the next 1/2 cup. Stir frequently, and continue adding the vegetable broth 1/2 cup at a time. A lot of chefs advise keeping the vegetable broth heating on the stove so that it

is already simmering and hot when you add it to the rice.

3. Once you've added all the vegetable broth and the rice is nearly cooked, add in the canned pumpkin, fresh ginger, nutmeg, fresh basil and vegan margarine or butter. Stir well to mix everything well, and season lightly with a bit of salt and pepper.

4. All everything to heat, just for another minute or two, until everything is thoroughly heated through, and stirring frequently.

Vegan Cream of Broccoli Soup

Ingredients:

- 3 cups broccoli (florets)
- 1 cup broccoli (stems, chopped, thick skins removed)
- 1 1/2 cups water
- 2 tablespoons lemon juice (freshly squeezed)
- 1/2 cup cashews (raw)
- 1/2 cup celery (sliced)
- 1/4 cup onion (chopped yellow or red)
- Optional: 1 clove garlic
- 1 tablespoon dill (fresh or 1 teaspoon dried dill)
- 1 teaspoon rosemary (fresh or 1/2 teaspoon dried rosemary)
- 1 tablespoon parsley (fresh or 1 teaspoon dried parsley)
- 1 teaspoon thyme (fresh or 1/2 teaspoon dried thyme)
- 1 tablespoon nama shoyu
- 2 tablespoons yeast (nutritional)
- 1/2 teaspoon salt (sea)
- 1/2 teaspoon black pepper
- Optional: 1/4 teaspoon crushed red pepper or cayenne)
- 1/2 teaspoon celery seed

Instructions:

1. Place all of the ingredients in a blender and blend for 30 to 40 seconds or until a creamy consistency is reached. You may wish to add a little more water. Serve immediately. If refrigerated, you may want to warm the soup to room temperature before serving. Garnish your raw cream of broccoli soup with extra fresh dill.

Vegan Indian Cauliflower Curry

Ingredients:

- 1 1/2 teaspoon fresh ginger, grated
- 2 tablespoons sesame seeds
- 3 tablespoons peanuts
- 3 cloves garlic, minced
- 1 tablespoon cumin
- 1 teaspoon ground cloves
- 1 teaspoon turmeric
- 1/2 teaspoon cayenne pepper
- 2 tablespoon water
- 1 tablespoon vegetable oil
- 2 onions, diced
- 1 cauliflower, chopped
- 1 1/2 tablespoon lemon juice

Instructions:

1. In a blender or food processor, grind together the ginger, sesame seeds, peanuts, garlic, spices, and water.
2. Sautee the onions in vegetable oil in a pan over medium-high heat, about three to five minutes, or until onions turn clear.
3. Add the cauliflower and spices mixture to the pan and cover it.

4. Allow to cook another 10 to 12 minutes, occasionally stirring until cauliflower is almost fully cooked.
5. Add lemon juice and allow to cook for 3 more minutes.
6. Enjoy as a side dish or pair with Indian naan for a warming and nourishing meal.

SMOOTHIES

AND

SNACKS

Sweet Pineapple Smoothie

Ingredients:

- ½ cup pineapple
- ½ ripe mango, cut in cubes
- 1 ripe banana, quartered (preferably frozen)
- 1/3 cup orange juice
- 3-4 ice cubes

Instructions:

1. Place all the ingredients in the blender, blend until smooth. Then serve in a nice tall glass.

Four Berries Smoothie

Ingredients:

- 10 pcs of blueberries
- 1 cup fresh orange juice or grapefruit juice
- 6 pcs strawberries
- 1 large banana, peeled
- 4 pcs blackberries
- 1 fresh dates
- 4 pcs raspberries

Instructions:

1. Put all the ingredients in a speed blender and food processor and process until smooth. Serve and enjoy.

Green Mango Smoothie

Ingredients:

- 2 pcs mangoes, peeled and diced
- 2 cups of spinach
- 1-2 cup coconut water or alternative with plain water

Instructions:

1. Put all the ingredients in a blender or food processor and blend or process until smooth. Add water or coconut water on your desired consistency. Serve and enjoy.

Raspberry Kale Green Smoothie

Ingrdients:

- ½ cup chopped kale
- 2 leaves kale
- ½ ripe banana
- 1 cup sliced cucumber
- 3-4 ice cubes

Instructions:

1. Blend all the ingredients in a blender until smooth. Serve and enjoy.

Triple Berry Smoothie

Ingredients:

- 1 ripe banana
- ½ cup chopped strawberries
- ½ cup blueberries
- ½ cup blackberries
- 1 1/2 cups chopped spinach
- 1/2 cup unsweetened soy milk
- 1 tablespoon ground chia seeds

Instructions:

1. Place all ingredients in blender and blend until smooth.it can beserve over ice.

Papaya and Banana Smoothie

Ingredients:

- 3 ice cubes
- 1 cup papaya, chopped
- ½ cup fresh orange juice
- 2 pcs ripe bananas
- 3 pcs of kale leaves, chopped
- 1/4 cup chopped cucumber

Instructions:

1. Blend all ingredients together in a blender until smooth. Serve and enjoy.

Coconut and Green-Tea Smoothie

Ingredients:

- 2 leaves of kale
- ½ cup shredded coconut
- 1 tsp agave nectar
- ½ of green tea
- 2- 3 ice cubes

Instructions:

1. Place all ingredients in a blender, blend until smooth. Serve and enjoy.

Orange Carrot Smoothie

Ingredients:

- 2 cups of chopped kale
- 1 cup of chopped carrots
- 1 cup fresh orange juice
- 3 ice cubes

Instructions:

1. Combine all ingredients in the blender, blend until smooth. Serve and enjoy.

Cranberry and Raspberry Smoothie

Ingredients:

- ½ cup fresh cranberries
- ½ chopped cucumber
- ½ cup fresh raspberries
- 1 tsp hemp seeds
- ½ cup of water
- 5 pcs ice cubes

Instructions:

1. Put all the ingredients in the blender and blend until smooth. Serve and enjoy.

Plum Celery Smoothie

Ingredients:

- 1 1/2 cup non-dairy milk
- 1 cup pitted and chopped plums
- 1 cup celery
- ½ cup lettuce
- 1 tsp vanilla extract
- 1 tablespoon chia seed
- 3 pcs ice cubes

Instructions:

1. Combine all ingredients in the blender and blend until smooth. Serve and enjoy.

Blueberry Banana Peach Smoothie

Ingredients:

- 1/2 peach, chopped
- 1 cup blueberries
- 1 cup kale
- 1 cup watercress
- 1 tablespoon flax seeds
- 1 banana, frozen, quartered

Instructions:

1. Combine all ingredients in the blender until it is well blended and serve it fresh as it tends to change color in time.

Avocado and Banana Smoothie

Ingredients:

- 1 ripe banana
- 1 ripe avocado
- 2 cups of almond milk
- 4 pcs of pitted dates
- 2 tablespoons chia seeds
- 2 tablespoons maple syrup or corn syrup
- A pinch of cinnamon powder

Instructions:

1. Combine all ingredients in the blender until it is well blended and serve it fresh as it tends to change color in time.

Avocado Mint Smoothie

Ingredients:

- ½ ripe avocado, peeled
- 2 cups of almond milk
- 2 pcs mint leaves
- 2 tablespoons agave syrup
- ½ cup of plain yogurt
- ½ cup crushed ice

Instructions:

1. Put all the ingredients together in a blender and blend until smooth. Serve the smoothie fresh as it tends to change color in time.

Celery Apple Smoothie

Ingredients:

- 1 stalk of celery, chopped
- 2 pcs kale leaves
- 2 pcs of green apples, sliced
- A pinch of cinnamon powder
- 2 tablespoons of raw honey
- 1 lime, zested and juiced
- 1 cup of plain yogurt
- 4 ice cubes

Instructions:

1. Combine all ingredients in the blender until it is well blended and serve it fresh as it tends to change color in time.

Almond Strawberry Smoothie

Ingredients:

- 1 cup of almond milk
- ¼ cup of almonds, blanched
- 1 cup fresh spinach
- 1 cup of fresh strawberries
- 1 tablespoon of raw honey
- ½ ripe banana
- 1 tsp lemon juice
- 4 ice cubes

Instructions:

1. Combine all ingredients in the blender until it is well blended and serve it fresh as it tends to change color in time.

Watermelon Spinach Smoothie

Ingredients:

- 2 cups of fresh spinach
- ¼ cup of coconut cream
- 1 cup of seedless watermelon cut in cubes
- 1 cup of coconut water
- 1 tablespoon lemon juice
- 2 pcs of mint leaves
- 4 ice cubes

Instructions:

1. Combine all ingredients in the blender until it is well blended and serve it fresh as it tends to change color in time.

Peach Coconut Smoothie

Ingredients:

- 1 cup of vanilla ice cream
- 5 slices of large peaches
- 1 can of organic coconut milk
- 2 tsp of pure vanilla extract
- 1 tablespoon of agave nectar
- 1 cup of water

Instructions:

1. Wash and slice the peaches and remove the seeds. Then mix all the ingredients together in a blender and blend until smooth. Serve and enjoy.

Banana and Papaya Smoothie

Ingredients:

- 1 cup coconut water
- 1 ripe banana, peeled
- 1 cup papaya, chopped
- ½ cup of chopped cucumber
- 1/2 cup celery
- 1 tablespoon almond

Instructions:

1. Combine all ingredients together in a blender until smooth. Serve and enjoy.

Apple Cinnamon with

Spinach Smoothie

Ingredients:

- 1 cup of non-dairy milk
- 2 cups of spinach
- 1 apple, chopped
- 1/8 tsp of pure vanilla extract
- ¼ tsp ground cinnamon
- 2-3 ice cubes

Instructions:

1. Place all ingredients in a blender and blend until smooth. Serve and enjoy

Banana Spinach Smoothie

Ingredients:

- 1 cup of spinach
- 1 cup of almond milk
- 1 frozen banana

Instructions:

1. Mix all ingredients in a blender and blend until smooth. Serve and enjoy.

Caramel Peanut Butter Fudge Brownies

Ingredients:

- 2 (8-inch) boxes brownie mix
- 1/2 cup peanut butter
- 11 tablespoons water
- 1/4 cup oil
- 2 eggs
- 1 cup brown sugar
- 1 cup corn syrup
- 1-1/4 cups peanut butter
- 2 cups chocolate chips (semisweet)
- 1/3 cup peanut butter

Instructions:

1. Preheat oven to 350 degrees F. Grease 13" x 9" pan with nonstick baking spray and set aside.
2. Combine brownie mix in a large bowl, 1/2 cup of peanut butter, water, oil, and eggs; mix until blended, then beat 30 strokes. Pour into prepared pan. Bake for 35-45 minutes or until brownies are just set; do not over bake. Let cool on wire rack.
3. In medium microwave-safe bowl, combine brown sugar and corn syrup.

4. Microwave mixture on high heat for 2 minutes,
    then remove and stir. Return to microwave and
    cook on high heat for 1-1/2 minutes longer.
5.   Remove from microwave and immediately stir
    in 1-1/4 cups peanut butter. Mix well with wire
    whisk and quickly pour over cooled brownies.
    Spread evenly to cover.
6.   Combine chocolate chips and 1/3 cup of
    peanut butter in a small microwave-safe bowl.
    Microwave on high for 1-1/2 minutes, then
    remove and stir until chips melt and mixture is
    smooth.

Pour the caramel mixture on and carefully, with the back of a spoon, spread evenly over the caramel mixture. Let stand until set, then cut into bars.

Chocolate Cake

Ingredients:

- 1 ¾ cup flour
- ¾ cups unsweetened cocoa powder
- 1 ½ tsp. baking powder
- 1 ½ tsp. baking soda
- ¼ tsp. salt
- 1 12.3-ounce box firm silken tofu
- 1 1/4 cup maple syrup
- 3 Tbsp. canola oil
- 1 cup almond milk
- 1/3 cup water (boiling)

Instructions:

1. Preheat the oven to 350 F. Lightly oil or grease (with dairy-free soy margarine) two 9" round cake pans. Set aside.
2. In a medium-sized mixing bowl, sift together the flour, cocoa powder, baking powder, baking soda and salt. Set aside.
3. In a blender, process the tofu until creamy. Add maple syrup and oil and blend until smooth. Stir the tofu mixture and almond milk into the dry ingredients. Add the boiling water and continue to stir until the batter is well blended. (The batter should be smooth but with some lumps in it.)

4. Pour the batter on the prepared pans and bake
    for at least 25-30 minutes, or until a toothpick
    inserted into the center of the cakes comes out
    clean. Let the cakes to cool in the pans for at
    least 15-20 minutes on a wire cooling rack
    before removing from the pans to finish cooling
    on the cooling rack. Once cakes are
    completely cool, frost with dairy-free frosting of
    your choice.

Vegan Bruschetta

Ingredients:

- 12 slices French bread (or Italian bread, lightly toasted)
- 3 large tomatoes (chopped)
- 1 tablespoon olive oil
- 3 tablespoons fresh basil (chopped)
- 1/4 teaspoon sea salt (or kosher salt)
- Dash fresh cracked pepper

Instructions:

1. Chop the tomatoes. You may want to remove excess seeds and pulp.
2. Chop the fresh basil.
3. Combine the tomatoes, oil, basil, and salt in a covered bowl and let marinate at least 4 hours. Do not refrigerate as the tomatoes will lose their flavor in the refrigerator.
4. Immediately before serving, toast the bread slices lightly.
5. Use a spoon with slots to layer the tomato basil mixture onto bread.
6. Crack fresh pepper over the top. Serve immediately.
7. Bruschetta will be paired well with other Italian dishes for a meal.

Baked Healthy Cinnamon Sugar Tortilla Chips

Ingredients:

- 4 flour tortillas
- 2 tbsp. vegan margarine, melted
- 1 tbsp. cinnamon
- 1 tbsp. sugar

Instructions:

1. Slice the flour tortillas like a pizza into 6 slices to create tortilla "chips".
2. Drizzle each tortilla "chips" with melted margarine and then sprinkle with cinnamon and sugar.
3. Bake at 350 F for at least 10 minutes, or until desired crispiness is reached.
4. Serve with fresh fruit salsa or just snack on them and enjoy!
5. Tips and other variations:
6. If you're not a vegan, try a little honey butter and cinnamon instead of regular butter. Cut back the extra sugar in this case, as the honey butter is sweet enough on its own.
7. Here's how to fry these chips instead of baking:
1. Omit the vegan margarine and fry the flour tortillas in oil until crispy (for about 2 minutes),

then quickly coat with cinnamon and sugar.
Place the cinnamon and sugar in a bowl or in a
bag and then just gently toss to coat evenly
and well.

Easy and Homemade Guacamole

Ingredients:

- 1 large avocado (ripe)
- 1 tsp. lemon juice (or lime juice)
- 1/4 cup prepared salsa
- 1/4 tsp. garlic powder
- Dash salt to taste (sea salt or kosher salt is highly recommended)
- Optional: dash cayenne or chili powder (or about 1/2-1 tsp hot sauce or taco sauce)

Instructions:

1. First, make sure your avocado is just soft and ripe enough. If it isn't, you might want to check out a few tips for how to ripen avocados here.
2. Slice avocado in half and remove the pit. Scoop out the green part in a spoon into a small or medium-sized bowl.
3. Next, mash the avocado with a fork until almost smooth, or until desired consistency is reached. Generally, a few small chunks are ok, but it is mostly smooth.
4. When your avocado is already mashed, add the lemon or lime juice, the prepared salsa, garlic powder, the sea salt or kosher salt and the cayenne powder, chili powder, hot sauce,

or taco sauce, if you're using it. Gently mix it all
together until well blended.

5. You can adjust the seasonings to taste, or, just
   go ahead and dip your chips and enjoy your
   super easy guacamole with store-bought salsa!

Tips:

1. Guacamole doesn't keep well. It's best to
   prepare then serve the moment it is already
   prepared. Freshness is important when it
   comes to guacamole! If you have to store your
   guacamole in the fridge for a while, transfer it
   into as small a container and cover it to prevent
   it from going brown.

Vegan Mango Salsa with Peaches

Ingredients:

- 2 mangos, peeled and chopped
- 2 fresh peaches, peeled and chopped
- 1 medium sized sweet onion, diced
- 1 medium tomato, diced (optional)
- 2 cloves garlic, finely minced
- 2 tbsp chopped fresh cilantro
- juice of one lime
- dash salt and pepper

Instructions:

1. Combine all ingredients and chill. It is better if you have a food process so you can process all the ingredients in chunks, rather than dicing and chopping.
2. Chill before serving. Taste, and add a bit more salt and pepper, lime, or cilantro to taste.
3. Makes four servings of mango salsa.

Home Fried Sweet Potatoes

Ingredients:

- 1/3 cup canola oil
- 6 pcs large sweet potatoes, peeled and cubed
- 1 tsp salt
- 1/2 tsp garlic powder
- 1/2 tsp paprika

Instructions:

1. Use a large pan to heat canola oil over medium-high heat.
2. Add sweet potatoes and cook, stirring occasionally, until sweet potatoes are golden brown. Seasonit as desired with salt, pepper, garlic powder and paprika.
3. Let cool to desired temperature and serve.

Conclusion

After serving a palatable vegan dishes through this book, it is only on one's choice to what lifestyle should be chosen. But vegan or not, you can also prepare all the delectable dishes this book offers.

As long as it doesn't compromise anyone's health, variety of food can be enjoyed but all in moderation and self-discipline.

About The Author

The Health Buff is a group of writers that aims to help people on what diet they want to achieve. They explore a lot of dishes from different parts of the world and share them by putting everything into a book. These writers specifically share the diets and food that just actually worked for them.

The Health Buff writers are all food and health enthusiasts, thus, coming up with the idea of sharing what they all love to do to inspire other people look after their health. They all believed that the best investment that you can ever make is in your own HEALTH.

www.ingramcontent.com/pod-product-compliance
Lightning Source LLC
Chambersburg PA
CBHW060752260726
48660CB00002B/580